T0144840

# MAITAKE GOLD 404®

## THE ULTIMATE IMMUNE SUPERNUTRIENT

### Learn How This Medicinal Mushroom Formulation:

- Fights Cancer Four Ways
- Helps Detoxify the Body
- Helps Lower Cholesterol and High Blood Pressure
- Provides Cellular Protection and Enhances Immune Function

## Mark Stengler, N.D.

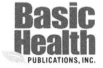

Basic Health
PUBLICATIONS, INC.

The information contained in this book is based upon the research and personal and professional experiences of the author. It is not intended as a substitute for consulting with your physician or other healthcare provider. Any attempt to diagnose and treat an illness should be done under the direction of a healthcare professional.

The publisher does not advocate the use of any particular healthcare protocol but believes the information in this book should be available to the public. The publisher and author are not responsible for any adverse effects or consequences resulting from the use of the suggestions, preparations, or procedures discussed in this book. Should the reader have any questions concerning the appropriateness of any procedures or preparation mentioned, the author and the publisher strongly suggest consulting a professional healthcare advisor.

Series Cover Designer: Mike Stromberg
Editor: Stephany Evans
Typesetter: Gary A. Rosenberg

Basic Health Guides are published by
**Basic Health Publications, Inc.**

# Contents

# Foreword

As an immunologist and a senior professor of microbiochemistry at Kobe Pharmaceutical University in Kobe, Japan, I have been researching medicinal mushrooms for more than twenty years. For the past fifteen years, I have focused exclusively on maitake mushrooms. The decision to focus specifically on this fine mushroom stemmed from my earlier research, through which I'd discovered that the maitake mushroom has the highest level of bioavailability (that is, the highest level of therapeutic activity) by oral administration of any medicinal mushroom. My research led me to discover what I named the "D fraction" extract, derived from maitake, which significant research has indicated has antitumor and immunopotentiating (immune-enhancing) activity. I have since discovered a most important advance on that original extract. The D fraction extract contained an inhibitory substance, or "float, that actually had anti-immunopotentiating action. By removing the float, the D fraction activity is improved by at least 30 percent. This new discovery was so significant that in 1998 I was awarded United States patent #5,854,404 on this development. This improved extract is known as "MD fraction" and is sold in North America under the name MaitakeGold 404®. This is the only maitake product based on my scientific research and my innovations in the field of medicinal mushrooms, and the only maitake product I endorse. I urge readers of this book to look for the MaitakeGold 404® name on any maitake product that they purchase to insure they are getting the highest quality maitake extract.

I am very pleased that health professionals such as Dr. Mark Stengler are spreading the word on MaitakeGold 404® and its importance in the treatment of serious health issues such as cancer, as well as the vital role it can play as an everyday immunopotentiator (immune enhancer) and cellular protectant. MaitakeGold 404® should be taken every day, along with multi-vitamins and antioxidants, to protect cellular health and prevent against illness down the road. I have seen MaitakeGold 404® extract touch many lives in a positive healing way, and it is my sincerest hope that in reading this book you'll be inspired to make MaitakeGold 404® a part of your personal health regimen. Let MaitakeGold 404® help you reach your good health goals.

—Professor Hiroaki Nanba, Ph.D.

# Introduction

The statistics are sobering. According to the American Cancer Society, men have about a one in two lifetime risk of developing cancer; women have about a one in three risk. Cancer is the second leading cause of death in North America next to heart disease. More than 1,500 Americans die each day from cancer.[1] With statistics like these, it is no wonder health conscious consumers are seeking nontoxic, natural therapies that will assist their bodies in preventing as well as battling cancer. However, it is often difficult for consumers to separate fact from fiction, or real hope from hype, with the myriad of natural products available that claim cancer-fighting benefits.

In addition, an increasingly toxic environment has placed a great burden on the cellular defenses of our bodies. As a result, many are in need of extra nutritional support to maintain a healthy immune system. Without a healthy defense system, one opens the floodgates to disease and poor vitality. A large percentage of the general public—as well as concerned doctors like myself—is availing itself of the best of what nature has to offer in order to live life to its fullest. The sheer number of nutritional products that fill health food store shelves is often overwhelming. There is one product, however, I have come to view as standing above all others: MaitakeGold 404®.

This powerful ally in the battle against cancer and many other diseases is derived from the maitake (*my-TAH-key*) mushroom. So impressive is the science behind MaitakeGold 404® that one of the world's most respected cancer institutes was awarded a $500,000 grant to conduct research on MaitakeGold 404® and its effects on breast cancer patients. This book will provide the information needed to understand what MaitakeGold 404® is, the scientific data that stands behind it, how it works, its safety record, and how best to use it both preventatively and therapeutically.

# 1. What Is Maitake?

**M**aitake as translated in Japanese means "dancing mushroom." There are several different explanations as to how it came to be named. One is that in ancient Japan, people would dance with joy when they found maitake because it was so valuable and costly. Another version suggests that this overjoyed dance was because maitake is so delicious and healthful. Another explanation is that the fruiting bodies of clustered maitake overlap one another and resemble butterflies in a wild dance.[2,3]

The botanical name for maitake is *Grifola* ("braided fungus") *frondosa* ("leaf like"). The mature mushroom has overlapping, large fleshy grayish-brown caps so is also sometimes referred to as "Hen of the Woods," as it resembles the backside of a hen. Maitake grows in the forests of Asia, Europe, Canada, and parts of the Eastern United States. It grows in heavy clumps (sometimes 100 pounds or more) at the base of stumps and on the roots of trees. Indigenous to Northern Japan, maitake has long been a highly valued edible mushroom, described as having a meaty taste. One can often find it for sale in natural health grocery stores and Asian markets.

## A HISTORICAL PERSPECTIVE

For thousands of years, potent medicinal actions of specific mushrooms that can help humans prevent and recover from illness have been recorded. Medicinal mushrooms have long been revered in Asia and other areas of the world for their many healing benefits. Ancient Japanese and Chinese medical texts describe the medicinal properties of various mushrooms. Some of the earliest recorded uses of maitake were described in the *Shen Nong Ben Cao Jing*, the Chinese Materia Medica from the Han dynasty (206 B.C.–220 A.D.). These included the treatment of stomach problems and hemorrhoids, calming the mind and nerves, and improving the function of the spleen (the spleen in Chinese medicine refers to a digestive organ that is intricately tied into the immune system).[4]

The Japanese have long used maitake as an adaptogen, a nutrient that helps to balance the various systems and functions of the body.

Popular medicinal mushroom extracts from Asia include those derived from shiitake, reishi, and kawaratake. These extracts are used for their immune-enhancing effects for conditions such as cancer, HIV, hepatitis, chronic fatigue syndrome, and other immune-related conditions. In the past decade, as the result of studies released on its immune-potentiating and anti-cancer activity, interest in maitake, above other types of medicinal mushrooms, has skyrocketed. In Japan, maitake has long been recognized as the "King of the Mushrooms," and has held a special status among medicinal mushrooms. In fact, maitake was so revered in Japan that collectors would keep the forest locations of their mushroom-gathering grounds a secret.

Up until 1979, maitake was harvested only in the wild. Since then, Japanese cultivation of maitake for distribution as a food and dietary supplement has been steadily increasing for worldwide export. Cultivation has made it possible to produce maitake in large enough quantities that now people around the world can enjoy the benefits of this important mushroom extract.

Currently, MaitakeGold 404® extract is a popular therapy for cancer and hepatitis in Japan and around the world. It has also shown some promise in treating hypertension, high cholesterol and triglycerides, weight loss, diabetes, malaria, chronic fatigue syndrome, HIV, and other chronic viral infections.

# 2. The Evolution of MaitakeGold 404®

In the early 1980s, Dr. Hiroaki Nanba, a professor of microbiology and expert mycologist at Kobe Pharmaceutical University, was intensively studying the medicinal properties of various mushrooms. During this time, much of his attention was devoted to the popular shiitake mushroom. However, when his research showed him that maitake had a unique molecular structure that exhibited greater antitumor activity than other mushroom extracts he had been working with, his attention was diverted. Maitake, he discovered, also was unique in that it showed the greatest effectiveness of any mushroom when given orally. This action was extremely important as most clinical studies on mushroom extracts had so far found injection to be the most efficacious route of administration. At this point, Dr. Nanba decided to devote his focus exclusively on maitake.

## MAITAKE D FRACTION

Dr. Nanba worked with other Japanese scientists to extract various polysaccharides (high molecular weight compounds of connecting sugars) from maitake and to test them for anticancer properties and for their potential as immunomodulators. An immunomodulator is a substance that enhances the body's natural defense system or one that brings the immune system back into balance.

In 1984, Dr. Nanba discovered an important maitake fraction (or specialized component) that stimulated macrophages, the white blood cells that are essential to a powerful immune system. Through a special extraction method, the important "D fraction," as it was named, was isolated. It was now possible to produce a standardized form of specific beta-glucan polysaccharides—beta-1,6 glucan and beta-1,3 glucan. (See the inset "Beta-Glucans" on page 11.) Dr. Nanba patented this D fraction that same year. This iso-lation and extraction method of the D fraction was important as it now enabled one to focus on the components (specific beta-glucans) that improved immune function. It also allowed for more concentrated products to be developed so that massive quantities of the medicinal substance would not need to be ingested orally for a therapeutic response.

Other herbal products or foods also contain polysaccharides and beta-glucans. But the type of beta-glucans is important in regard to immune function. Dr. Nanba found that maitake D fraction's unique beta-glucan structure has more branching chains than other mushroom extracts: it is thought that the more branching chains there are, the more potential there is that immune cells will be activated. So because of its unique configuration, as well as the fact that it has a high molecular weight, D fraction is believed to activate many immune cells, that is, more than other mushroom extracts. In a 1995 study published in the *New York Academy of Sciences,* Dr. Nanba is quoted as saying, "I have been involved in research on the medicinal properties of edible mushrooms for the last 15 years and have reported that, of all medicinal mushrooms studied, maitake mushroom (*Grifola frondosa*) has the strongest antitumor activity and tumor growth inhibition both when administered orally and intraperitoneally [injection into the abdomen cavity]."[5] The D fraction was then shown in animal studies to stop the metastasis (spread) of cancer cells as well as to prevent cancer formation in normal cells.[6] Maitake fractions seem to have a specific antitumor action, potentially slowing the growth of tumors in the breast, colon, lungs, stomach, liver, prostate, brain, and other organs.

## BEYOND THE D FRACTION—MD FRACTION

Dr. Nanba continued his research on the D fraction in order to provide an even larger amount of the key compound for use in dietary supplements. His diligence paid off, and in 1996, he was awarded a Japanese Patent on an advanced form of the D fraction, which was named the MD fraction. By adding a step to the extraction process—a further purification of the D fraction whereby floating or adhering matter is removed—he was able to create the purest and most bioactive form of the D fraction. Thus, as the MD fraction patent describes, "Because removal of the floating and adhering matter brings about an enhancement in the antitumor activity and immunopotentiating activity of the extract, the step of removing said matter is extremely important."[7] Tests on the MD fraction have shown a superior effect in regard to antitumor and immunopotentiating activity. For example, tumors in mice were shown to be significantly more inhibited by the MD fraction when compared with the D fraction. The MD fraction also demonstrated a much more favorable effect on macrophages and killer T cells than that of the D fraction.[8] It is this fraction that is found in MaitakeGold 404®, the preferred form of maitake as Dr. Nanba's research has demonstrated. In later chapters, I will discuss more in depth how MaitakeGold 404® extract improves immune status, protects cells against toxins and free radicals, and how it fights cancer and reduces the side effects of chemotherapy.

MaitakeGold 404® extract is a trademarked product (US patent #5,854,404). "404" in the product name refers to the last three number of this patent. This product is the only source of the MD fraction.

## MAITAKE MUSHROOMS VERSUS MAITAKEGOLD 404®

Maitake mushrooms are a popular and nutritious culinary delicacy found in world-class restaurants around the world. They are also available commercially for home use and are popular in many homes in North America. However, for therapeutic effects on the immune system, maitake mushroom as a food does not compare to that of maitake supplements such as MaitakeGold 404®. Maitake mushrooms can be eaten and supplemented on a daily basis for optimal immune function. For those with serious diseases such as cancer or hepatitis, it is imperative that maitake be taken in the supplement form.

# 3. A Golden Remedy for the Immune System

To understand how MaitakeGold 404® affects the immune system, it is important first to review the mechanics of this elaborate system. There are two types of immunity in the human body: cellular immunity and humoral immunity. These two components of the immune system protect us from anything foreign to the body, including infectious agents and foreign particles.

## CELLULAR IMMUNITY

In cellular immunity, the essential player in the first line of defense are the white blood cells called macrophages ("large eaters"). The macrophage is the largest of the white blood cells and is the immune cell responsible for phagocytosis (the process of killing or destroying pathogens and cancerous cells). Macrophages also have the important responsibility of regulating the immune system and are considered among the most active and important agents of the immune system.

White blood cells called T lymphocytes (or T cells) identify and then destroy cancerous cells, viruses, and microorganisms like fungi and bacteria. T lymphocytes grow and mature in the thymus gland (hence the T prefix) and are responsible for the development of specific immunities. They are released into the bloodstream to seek out and destroy antigens (substances that cause an immune response), which can range from benign substances such as pollen to more harmful substances such as bacteria, partly through the secretion of proteins called cytokines (such as Interferon).

B cells (which are also white blood cells) from bone marrow, produce antibodies, and natural killer, or NK, cells (specialized white blood cells) that destroy infected or cancerous cells in the body.

The following immune cells play a role in fighting cancer and infections:

- Macrophages—devour cancer cells and pathogens. In doing so, they stimulate the activity of other immune cells.

- Neutrophils—fight infections and cancer cells and destroy waste matter. They comprise 60 to 70 percent of all white blood cells.

- Lymphocytes—flow inside lymphatic vessels, blood, and between tissues. They comprise 20 to 40 percent of all white blood cells. They include:
  - T helper cells—help assist other cells to destroy cancer cells.
  - Cytotoxic T cells—destroy cancer cells and viruses and other foreign matter.
  - B cells—produce antibodies that work on behalf of other immune cells to target cancer and other foreign invaders.
  - T suppressors—suppress excessive immune function.
  - Natural killer cells—As the name implies, these immune cells are designed to seek and destroy cancer and viruses. More independent than other cells, natural killer cells survey the body for "foreign invaders." Other members of the immune system will alert them to cancer cells and other intruders.

## HUMORAL IMMUNITY

Humoral immunity involves the production of antibodies. These are not cells, but rather special proteins whose chemical structures are shaped to match the surfaces of specific antigens. When they encounter their specific antigens, antibodies either damage the invasive cells or call white blood cells to attack. The immune system then files this antigen in its database so that if it ever encounters this antigen again, it knows how to defeat it. In this way, the inner workings of the immune system play a major role in disease prevention.

## FURTHER IMMUNE ACTIVITY

Various chemicals are also released by the immune system to arouse and increase immune activity. These include interferon (IFN), interleukin (IL), tumor necrosis factor (TNF), and killer cell activator. Maitake has been shown to increase the secretion of interleukin-1 and interleukin-2, which support the activity of cancer-fighting cells.

All of these different immune cells and chemicals work together to destroy cancer cells and infectious agents such as viruses, bacteria, fungus, and others. For example, when a macrophage comes into contact with a cancer cell, it releases tumor-necrotizing factor, which destroys cancer cells.

Simultaneously, the chemical interleukin-1 is produced. As a result, T helper cells are stimulated in their activity, which in turn activate natural killer cells and draw them toward the site of the cancer cell(s). Similar to a radar and missile system, B cells release antibodies that "tag" the cancer cell (or infectious agent) so that lymphocytes and other white blood cells are attracted to the diseased cell(s). In other words, the immune cells work together as a team through a cascade of events to optimize the "immune response."

## MAITAKE POTENTIATES THE IMMUNE SYSTEM

As previously noted, MaitakeGold 404® contains a unique type of beta-glucan. These molecules are often referred to as host defense potentiators (HDP) because of their ability to stimulate the natural defense mechanisms of the immune system. Specifically, maitake beta-glucans activate and enhance the actions of macrophages, natural killer cells, killer T cells, and killer cells, all of which attack cancer cells, viruses, and other harmful intruders. In addition, maitake beta-glucans also stimulate chemicals in the body that enhance immune substances such as interleukins (1 and 2) and lymphokines. This results in a potent defense mechanism within the body to prevent and fight off cancer and infections. Maitake fills a void in conventional medicine for nontoxic agents that kill cancer cells and viruses through immunomodulation. One study found that cancer cell-destruction activity was two to three times higher as a result of the administration of the MD fraction. According to studies, MD fraction has the ability to both directly enhance the damaging activity of NK cells against cancer cells and to change NK precursor cells into activated NK cells.[9]

## MAITAKE IMMUNE FACTORS

To understand why maitake contains these powerful immune-enhancing beta-glucans, we can look to the lifecycle of mushrooms. Mushrooms are near the bottom of the ladder in the ecosystem. They survive where not much else could, living on decayed material such as rotten wood and leaves in a hostile environment. During the mycelial stage (which is the time fungi spend most of their time actively digesting food and fighting competitors in the environment) in the mushroom lifecycle, digestive enzymes are excreted outside the cells, which work on cellulose and other material to break it down for food. Before the digested food can be absorbed, the mushroom must first deactivate any disease-causing germs or toxins by releasing special polysaccharides. So mushrooms such as maitake have their own immune system just as we humans do. Their survival depends on the efficiency of their immune system, as does our own survival depend on our immune system. Moreover, it has been discovered that maitake polysaccharides, when ingested by humans, are both compatible with, and also have a beneficial effect on, our human immune system.

Glucans found in medicinal mushrooms improve immune function by stimulating cell-mediated immunity. In this type of immune response, T cells, natural killer cells, and others increase in activity and number.

In addition to its unique molecular structure, which improves immune function, maitake contains an abundance of minerals, such as zinc, copper, potassium, as well as vitamin D and niacin (nicotinic acid).[10] It also contains important phospholipids (fatty substances), including phosphatidylcholine, phosphatidylethanolamine, phosphatidylinositol, and phosphatidylserine, that contribute to the health of cellular membranes.[11]

The special glucan structure in MD fraction (MaitakeGold 404® extract) has a unique design that allows it to be efficiently assimilated when taken orally. Other mushroom extracts, such as lentinan, the extract from the shitake mushroom (which along with maitake is also very popular in Japan as an anticancer agent) must be injected to be optimally effective.

## MAINTAINING IMMUNITY FOR CANCER PROTECTION

It is imperative that those who presently have cancer optimize their immune function to its fullest potential. No matter what type of therapy a person currently is receiving (for example, chemotherapy, radiation, or nutritional), he or she can only benefit from immune enhancement that will power the highly specialized immune cells to work to fight and eliminate cancer. Good nutri-

---

### BETA-GLUCANS

Studies have shown that various beta-glucans enhance the immune response. One example is purified beta-glucans from common bakers yeast (*Saccharomyces cerevisiae*). One can also find beta-glucans in certain foods such as oats and barley, although these kinds do not have much effect on the immune system (they can, however, help lower cholesterol and blood sugar levels). The unique beta-glucan structure of MaitakeGold 404® is one of the most powerful ways to naturally activate the immune system.

tion, including effective supplements, stress reduction, and positive imagery all contribute to providing our bodies and immune systems with what they need to fight cancer. The same approach can be used by those with a history of cancer or those who have a strong genetic susceptibility to cancer.

Many health professionals and healthy lifestyle consumers rely on MaitakeGold 404® not only for cancer prevention and adjunctive treatment, but also as a daily supplement for optimal health and function. Following are some key prophylactic, or preventive, uses of maitake that can make a difference in people's lives.

## Cellular Protection from Free-Radical Damage

Our bodies are subject to ongoing encounters with a multitude of toxins. Toxic metals, such as arsenic, lead, cadmium, and mercury, as well as pesticides, secondhand smoke, and food preservatives, all contribute to the formation of free radicals, a primary cause of cellular damage. Loosely defined, a free radical is a highly reactive molecule that can destroy body tissues, especially cell membranes. Some are the result of exposure to chemical pollutants, cigarette smoke, or even sunlight. But free radicals also are a natural byproduct of the cell's own metabolic activity. Your cells need to burn oxygen to produce their endless supply of life-giving chemicals. However, in the process, approximately 15 percent of the oxygen you breathe combines with fats and other substances to produce free radicals.

Free radicals damage cellular structures including DNA, so the cumulative damage they cause leads to cellular aging, as well as to many diseases including the two biggest killers of Americans, heart disease and cancer. Most carcinogens (cancer-causing compounds) act to produce free-radical or oxidative damage to cell structures.

Antioxidants, in contrast, are compounds that protect against free-radical damage. By mopping up free radicals, antioxidants prevent cancer and other degenerative diseases. They also slow down the aging process, enhance immune function, reduce inflammation, and fight allergies. Human cells contain an array of antioxidant enzymes as well as enzymes to repair damage to cellular components, including DNA-repair enzymes.

One can protect cellular immunity with vitamin C, selenium, carot-enoids, and several other antioxidants. Along with these, maitake and other medicinal mushrooms are valuable supplements for protecting cellular health. As discussed, these mushroom extracts enhance macrophage and other immune cell activity that promotes detoxification and repair in the body. Thus, MaitakeGold 404® works to clean up the toxins in the body that

## PREVENTING ILLNESS WITH MAITAKE

A healthy functioning immune system is critical to remaining disease free. Without our even being aware of it, our immune system is destroying cancer cells on a daily basis. In addition, immune cells are on constant surveillance for invading intruders such as viruses, bacteria, fungi, parasites, and a host of infectious organisms. This battle with cancer cells and microbes is one for which your immune system is designed and is able to handle. However, diet, lifestyle, environmental toxins, stress, and other factors (many of which are controllable) tend to suppress immune function. It is easier to prevent cancer or serious infections than to treat them. Maitake is one of the better supplements to take on a regular basis to support immune function as well as to promote detoxification.

contribute to cell DNA damage. As do antioxidants, maitake provides both cellular protection and immune system optimization.

## Maitake as Adaptogen

The likelihood of illness dramatically decreases when one's immune system can adapt to the stressors one is encountering. Maitake is also highly valued by natural health-care practitioners as an adaptogen (an agent for bringing the body back into balance). Because high dosages of MaitakeGold 404® are not required for this adaptogenic effect, unlike some popular immune-stimulating herbs used by consumers and health professionals, which can dangerously stress the body, maitake can be used on a long-term basis for immune-system enhancement and balance.

# 4. Cancer: An Overview of a Prevention Strategy

**C**ancer is a major health threat today and is projected to become the number one killer in the following decades. Healthy cells in the human body divide at a controlled rate so that dying cells can be replaced in a balanced manner, so, simply defined, cancer is the uncontrolled growth of abnormal cells. With cancer, cell division becomes unregulated and as a result tumors can form. A tumor can be benign or malignant.

A benign tumor is not cancerous and rarely dangerous. They usually can be removed, and in most cases, they do not come back. Cells from benign tumors do not spread to other parts of the body. Most important, benign tumors are not life threatening.

A malignant tumor is cancerous, in that the cells that comprise these tumors are abnormal. They divide without control or order, and they can invade and damage nearby tissues and organs. A malignant tumor may pose a major threat to one's health or life as it robs the body of nutrients and interferes with organ function. A malignant tumor can also metastasize (spread) to other areas of the body and invade other tissues. Cancer cells can break away from a malignant tumor and enter the bloodstream or the lymphatic system, spreading from the original (primary) cancer site to form new tumors in other organs.

## TYPES OF CANCER

**Carcinomas** are malignant tumors that begin in the lining layer (epithelial cells) of organs. Carcinomas account for at least 80 percent of all cancers.

**Sarcomas** are malignant tumors growing from connective tissues, such as cartilage, fat, muscle, or bone.

**Leukemias** are cancers involving the blood and blood-forming organs (bone marrow, lymphatic system, and spleen). Leukemias do not usually form a tumor; instead, these cancer cells circulate in the blood and through other tissues where they can accumulate.

# WHAT CAUSES CANCER?

The development of cancer is the result of damage to the genetic material that controls cellular function. Our genes are composed of molecules of deoxyribonucleic acid (DNA). DNA contains four building-block molecules known as nucleotides arranged in a double-helix (twisted ladder-like structure). The exact sequence of nucleotides of DNA provides the genetic code that gives orders to all human cells. When DNA becomes damaged by mutations (changes or mistakes in genes), it can lead to the death of the cell or loss of cellular control and the development of cancerous cells. The cause of damage to DNA structure—that is, the cause of cancer—can be exposure to sunlight, harmful chemicals from the environment, viruses, or simply an inherited defect. Free-radical damage is a chief initiating factor in cancer development.

Although a family history of cancer carries with it increased risk, most cancer researchers agree that, as a sole cause, genetics is relatively insignificant (somewhere between 5 and 15 percent). Beyond this small percentage of cancers, which is strongly genetic in origin, most cancers are caused by largely controllable factors, such as nutrition, lifestyle, and environmental factors. One of the weaknesses of conventional medicine in preventing and treating cancer is that diet, lifestyle, stress, and the ability to rid the body of environmental toxins rarely are addressed in a comprehensive fashion. Yet these are the factors that are both most influential and most controllable in the prevention of cancer, as well as playing important roles in the recovery from cancer. Obviously, to reduce the risk of cancer, we all need to reduce free-radical formation in the body, limit exposure to dietary and environmental sources of free radicals, and increase our intake of antioxidant nutrients.

## Toxins

Environmental toxins can negatively affect the functioning of the immune system, as well as cellular health, and play a major role as causative factors of cancer. To give you an idea of the extent of our exposure to these contaminants, the Environmental Protection Agency estimated that between the years 1987 and 1994, American businesses released an estimated 2.2 billion pounds of toxins into the environment![12] Some toxins are easily avoided while steering clear of others is more challenging. Common examples include the following:

- **Pesticides and herbicides**—While each exposure to these may be incremental, over the course of a lifetime, one can be exposed to or ingest large amounts of pesticides, herbicides, and other toxic food preservatives. Always wash fruits and vegetables before consuming; when possible, grow or purchase organic foods.

- **Toxic metals**—Arsenic, cadmium, lead, mercury, nickel, and many other toxic metals that people are exposed to through contaminated water, food, air, workplace, or dental work are suspect in causing certain cancers. High levels of many of these toxic metals can certainly cause immune suppression while even small amounts can cause DNA damage and mutation. Industrial pollution has contributed greatly to our toxic metal burden.

- **Tobacco**—The most preventable cause of cancer is smoking. Tobacco smoke contains several cancer-causing agents, and this deadly addiction accounts for 40 to 50 percent of premature mortality in the Western world.

- **Alcohol**—A correlation between excessive consumption of alcohol and cancer of various organs such as the liver, esophagus, breast, and others has been well established.

- **Metabolites of poor digestion and elimination**—The old naturopathic philosophy that "death begins in the colon" has proven to be true to a great degree. Research has shown that toxic byproducts of poor digestion and elimination act as harmful toxins in the body.

- **Radiation**—Radiation in the form of proper amounts of sunlight is healthy to the immune system while overdose (or too much of a good thing) is the major cause of deadly malignant melanoma—cancer of the skin. Additionally, radiation from man-made sources is a known risk factor for different types of cancer, such as thyroid cancer, for example.

## DIET AND CANCER

A healthy diet is key to preventing most cancers. It is now scientifically established and well accepted that certain dietary practices either contribute to or inhibit many forms of cancer. As a protection from cancer, one of the most important dietary recommendations is to eat an assortment of fruits and vegetables. Detailed population studies have demonstrated beyond question a substantial protective role for fruits and vegetables in cancer prevention as they enhance the body's ability to process and eliminate toxic compounds. On the strength of this established scientific base, there has been considerable effort by the U.S. and Canadian governments to get people to eat more of these foods—ideally, at least five servings per day. Many cancer researchers now feel that seven to ten servings of fruits and vegetables a day provide even stronger protection against cancer.

The 5-A-Day for Better Health campaign began in 1992. Despite taking this message to grocery stores, classrooms, television, work sites, churches, and elsewhere, only about 10 percent of people in Canada and the United States actually achieve the five-a-day recommendation, and virtually no one is eating enough of the fruits and vegetables that actually are the most important in fighting cancer. To help you get on the right track, choose at least five servings* per day from the following list. Try not to double up (that is, don't eat two or more servings of the same fruit or vegetable, as it is important to eat a variety of both every day).

• Apples
• Berries (such as raspberries, strawberries, and blueberries)
• Bell peppers (red, green, orange, and yellow)
• Broccoli
• Brussels sprouts
• Carrots
• Cauliflower
• Celery
• Cucumber
• Grapes
• Green beans
• Mangoes
• Melons (such as honeydew, watermelon, and cantaloupe)
• Onions and scallions
• Oranges
• Peaches and nectarines
• Pears
• Peas
• Squash (such as zucchini, pumpkin, and butternut)
• Tomato paste or juice
• Yams and sweet potatoes

*Serving size equals 1 medium fruit or $1/2$ cup of small or cut-up fruit; $3/4$ cup (180 milliliters) of 100 percent juice; $1/4$ cup dried fruit; $1/2$ cup raw non-leafy or cooked vegetables; 1 cup raw leafy vegetables (such as lettuce); $1/2$ cup cooked green beans or peas.

Another key dietary recommendation to lower cancer risk is to reduce the intake of meat and other animal foods. One of the most consistent findings in studies looking at diet and cancer is a positive correlation between meat consumption and an incidence of cancer. In other words, the higher the intake of meat and other animal products, the higher the rate of cancer. There are several obvious reasons for this association. Meat lacks the antioxidant and phytochemicals (plant-based nutrients) that protect us from cancer, while it contains a lot of saturated fats and potentially carcinogenic compounds that can actually increase the risk of developing cancer. Examples of cancer-causing compounds in meat are not only the pesticide residues mentioned earlier, but also compounds known as heterocyclic amines and polycyclic aromatic hydrocarbons. These toxic compounds form when meat is grilled, fried, or broiled. The more well done the meat is prepared, the higher the level of heterocyclic amines. If eaten at all, limit intake of red meat to less than three ounces daily (three ounces is about the size of a deck of cards), and avoid consuming well-done, charbroiled, and fat-laden meats, as well as cured meats like ham, hot dogs, bacon, and jerky.

## STAY ACTIVE AND FIT

Regular exercise has been shown to improve immune status and prevent many types of cancer. Thirty minutes or more of moderate exercise, five or more days a week, is recommended. Exercise will also help you stay within your healthy weight range, which is important for overall health. Being consistent with your exercise is important, so find a combination of exercises that you like to do. That way, it will be less likely that you'll become bored and slack off or quit.

## HAVE REGULAR CANCER CHECKUPS

Regular screening examinations by a health-care professional are very important in the battle against cancer. The earlier a cancer is discovered, the more likely that treatment will be successful. Over half of all new cancer cases involve cancers that can be caught early through a regular physical exam. These include cancers of the breast, colon, rectum, cervix, prostate, testes, oral cavity, and skin. (See the inset on the following page.)

# SUMMARY OF AMERICAN CANCER SOCIETY RECOMMENDATIONS FOR THE EARLY DETECTION OF CANCER

**Cancer-Related Checkup.** A cancer-related checkup is recommended every three years for people ages twenty to forty and every year for people ages forty and older. This exam should include health counseling and, depending on a person's age, might include examinations for cancers of the thyroid, oral cavity, skin, lymph nodes, testes, and ovaries, as well as for some nonmalignant diseases.

**Breast.** Women ages forty and older should have an annual mammogram, an annual clinical breast examination (CBE) by a health-care professional, and should perform monthly breast self-examinations. The CBE should be conducted close to the scheduled mammogram. Women ages twenty to thirty-nine should have a CBE by a health-care professional every three years and should perform monthly breast self-examinations.

**Colon and Rectum.** Beginning at age fifty, men and women should follow one of the examination schedules below:

- A fecal occult blood test every year and a flexible sigmoidoscopy every five years.

- A colonoscopy every ten years.

- A double-contrast barium enema every five to ten years.

- A digital rectal exam should be done at the same time as sigmoidoscopy, colonoscopy, or double-contrast barium enema. People who are at moderate or high risk for colorectal cancer should talk with a doctor about a different testing schedule.

**Prostate.** The ACS recommends that beginning at age fifty, men who have a life expectancy of at least ten additional years, and younger men who are at high risk have both a prostate-specific antigen (PSA) blood test and a digital rectal examination annually. Men in high-risk groups, such as those with a strong familial predisposition (that is, two or more affected first-degree relatives) or black men, may begin at a younger age (that is, forty-five years).

**Uterus.** *Cervix:* All women who are or have been sexually active or who are eighteen and older should have an annual Pap test and pelvic examination. After three or more consecutive satisfactory examinations with normal findings, the Pap test may be performed less frequently. Discuss the matter with your physician.

*Endometrium:* Women at high risk for cancer of the uterus should have a sample of endometrial tissue examined when menopause begins.

# 5. MaitakeGold 404® and Cancer Therapy

While mainstream oncology slowly widens its focus on the use of nutritional and natural therapies, the obvious mainstays remain chemotherapy, radiation, surgery, and immune stimulants (mainly synthetic versions). Depending on the type of cancer, your doctor may recommend one or more of these therapies. For example, skin cancer surgically removed in the initial stages is 100 percent curable.

It is beyond the scope of this book to take an in depth look at each of these therapies, but I do want to point out that none of them address the underlying reason why one got cancer in the first place. That is, they can be reached for only after the fact, unlike the preventative, antioxidant effect of maitake, which can harness the power of your exceptionally sophisticated immune system—created especially to destroy cancer cells, among other things.

## CANCER TREATMENT PROTOCOL

Whether one is using one or more of these conventional approaches or none, natural, nontoxic therapies such as MaitakeGold 404® can optimize your immune response for the best possible outcome. For those undergoing chemotherapy, the supplementation of maitake should be taken to reduce side effects. It also helps to support white blood cell count, which can fall dangerously low during chemotherapy, and reduce one's susceptibility to a potentially fatal secondary infection. Maitake also works at a deeper level, arousing and potentiating the highly efficient cancer-fighting cells of your immune system.

Choosing a treatment protocol for cancer is an individual choice and there are those who for whatever reason(s) choose natural therapy as their sole treatment. In any event, MaitakeGold 404® extract should be considered an important part of a comprehensive protocol as numerous scientific studies have confirmed its ability to enhance immune function.

# THE FOUR-WAY MECHANISM OF MAITAKEGOLD 404®

Dr. Nanba and other researchers have identified four basic ways maitake beta-glucans can counter cancer: 1) by protecting healthy cells from becoming cancerous, 2) by helping to prevent metastasis, 3) by slowing or stopping tumor growth, and 4) by working in conjunction with chemotherapy. Each of these actions is discussed below.

## 1. By protecting healthy cells from becoming cancerous.

In one study, twenty-week-old mice were injected in the back once with the cancer-causing substance 3-MCA, methylcholanthrene. Beginning on the fifteenth day after the injection, ten of the mice were fed 0.2 mg of MD fraction for fifteen consecutive days. The other ten in the control group received saline solution. At the end of the thirty days, the number of mice with cancer was 30.7 percent in the maitake group and 93.2 percent in the control group. Dr. Nanba has noted that lentinan from shiitake extract also is effective against MCA-induced cancer, but only when given through intravenous (IV) injection.[13]

In another study, mice were exposed to the carcinogen N-butyl-N-butanolnitrosamine (BBN), known to cause bladder cancer, every day for eight weeks and then, excluding a control group of ten mice, were fed medicinal mushrooms—maitake, shiitake, and oyster mushrooms. All ten mice in the control group developed bladder cancer. Among the rest of the mice, all of the mushrooms significantly reduced the number of bladder cancers, with the maitake being the most effective—46.7 percent of the mice treated with maitake developed bladder cancer compared with 52.9 percent of those fed shiitake and 65 percent of those fed oyster mushrooms. In all, the mushroom extracts were shown to prevent a significant depression in lymphocyte and natural killer cell activity.[14]

## 2. By helping to prevent the spread (metastasis) of cancer from one area of the body to another.

In one study, researchers injected liver cancer into the rear footpad of mice. The footpad was then removed some forty-eight hours later. Mice were divided into three groups. The control group received normal feed, while two other groups received either whole maitake powder as 20 percent of their diet, or 1 mg per kilogram, of D fraction intraperitoneally (into abdomen cavity) ten times. After thirty days, mice were observed for tumor growth as a result of metastasis to the liver. In the control group, 100 percent of the animals showed metastasis. By comparison, the D fraction prevented 91.3 percent of that total, and the maitake-powder group 81.3 percent.[15]

### 3. By slowing or stopping tumor growth.

Animal studies have also shown maitake to slow or stop the growth of tumors. This has also been seen with humans in a clinical setting.

In one study, researchers implanted different types of tumor and cancer-causing cells in the armpit area of experimental male mice. After twenty-four hours, the researchers administered into the abdominal cavity 1 mg per kilogram per day of a purified polysaccharide fraction extracted from the maitake. On the twenty-fifth day after the tumor and cancerous cells were implanted, the solid tumors were removed and weighed to obtain a tumor growth inhibition ratio. The maitake fraction was found to cause significant tumor growth inhibition.[16]

In 1998, researchers at the University of Massachusetts at Amherst found that an extract of maitake had significant inhibitory activity against human cervical cancer and T4 leukemic cells. The researchers concluded that further studies were definitely warranted.[17]

### 4. By working in conjunction with chemotherapy to lessen its side effects, such as hair loss, pain, and nausea, and to boost its positive effects.

Chemotherapy, as the name implies, is the use of chemicals to destroy cancer cells. Unfortunately, while it can kill cancer cells, it also destroys normal cells. During treatment, high amounts of toxic metabolites can be formed, which need to be detoxified by the body. As a result, side effects are common. Maitake is becoming popular to not only support the immune system to fight cancer but also to lessen chemotherapy side effects. A survey of 671 patients showed that combining chemotherapy with maitake treatment can reduce adverse reactions as well as diminish the pain that comes with terminal stage cancer.[18]

Maitake also appears to make chemotherapy more effective. One study compared the effects of MD fraction extract and the chemotherapy drug mitomycin (MMC) on mice with cancer. The MD fraction alone inhibited tumor growth more effectively (80 percent) than MMC alone (45 percent). However, the most effective tumor inhibition was observed with the combination of these two substances with almost 98 percent inhibition. This is an interesting partnership as maitake supports immune function while the MMC directly kills tumor cells.[19]

In traditional Chinese medicine, maitake is said to be the best cleansing

## METASTASIS

A tumor is not the biggest concern when it comes to cancer. Metastasis, or the spreading of cancer cells, is the real culprit when it comes to fatality from this disease. Cancer cells can enter the bloodstream or lymphatic fluids and take hold in vital organs such as the liver. Most people die as the result of metastasis to distant organs rather than from damage that has occurred at the original tumor site. Nutritional supplements such as MaitakeGold 404® may provide protection against the spreading of cancer cells.

of the medicinal mushrooms through its detoxifying effects on two major organs of elimination—the liver and the lungs. This may also be a reason why maitake acts to reduce side effects when used by people undergoing chemotherapy where function of the liver—one of the most important organs of the immune system—can become compromised.

Statistically speaking, most people who have cancer receive some type of conventional therapy (for example, chemotherapy, radiation, or surgery). MaitakeGold 404® extract generally will be used as a complementary therapy. MaitakeGold 404® is not only safe to use alongside these conventional therapies, but I, along with thousands of other doctors, recommend that people with cancer do use it. For those undergoing chemotherapy, the supplementation of maitake will potentially reduce side effects.

Maitake also helps to support white blood cell count that can fall dangerously low during chemotherapy; reduces one's susceptibility to a fatal secondary infection; and arouses and potentiates the highly efficient cancer-fighting cells of the immune system.

## MD FRACTION: A POWERFUL CANCER FIGHTER

In one interesting study showing the anticancer effects of maitake MD fraction, mice transplanted with MM-46 carcinoma (breast tumor) were given either 0.5 mg per kilogram of MD fraction by intraperitoneal injection or 1.0 mg per kilogram of MD fraction orally for ten days. After the twentieth day, the solid tumor was removed and weighed. A 75 to 85 percent tumor regression was observed. The activities of natural killer cells, cytotoxic T cells, macrophages, and delayed-type hypersensitive T cells were increased to 1.23

to 2.5 times by MD fraction. In addition, the production of Interleukin-1 (IL-1) from macrophage and of Interleukin-2 (IL-2) from helper T cells were potentiated to 1.7 to 3.4 times normal.[20]

The MaitakeGold 404® extract (MD fraction) had a significantly stronger inhibitory effect on tumor growth than that of the group given the D fraction previously formulated by Dr. Nanba. And as expected, the MaitakeGold 404® extract exhibited greater immune-enhancing activity than the D fraction.[21] Table 5.1 below summarizes the effects on two key components of the immune system:

| TABLE 5.1. EFFECTS ON MACROPHAGES AND KILLER T CELLS | | |
| --- | --- | --- |
| | **Macrophages** | **Killer T Cells** |
| Control group (given physiological saline) | 100 percent | 100 percent |
| Group given substance A (D fraction extract) | 157.2 percent | 233.7 percent |
| Group given substance B (MaitakeGold 404®) | 203.5 percent | 284.5 percent |

## HUMAN STUDIES WITH MAITAKE MD FRACTION

Since MD fraction demonstrated beneficial effects against cancer in animals, a non-randomized clinical trial using MD fraction and maitake tablets (tablets contain whole herb maitake rather than the distilled fraction) was conducted to investigate a similar effectiveness with advanced cancer patients.

A total of thirty-three cancer patients in stages II, III, and IV, ages thirty-three to sixty-eight, participated in this trial; data was collected under the cooperation of their medical doctors in Japan. Patients were given either MD fraction with tablets only, or MD fraction and tablets in addition to chemotherapy. Cancer regression or significant symptom improvement was observed in eleven out of sixteen breast cancer patients, seven out of twelve liver cancer patients, and five out of eight lung cancer patients.[22]

Following are some case histories in which the MD fraction was used with advanced cancer patients. These have been excerpted from Dr. Nanba's book *Maitake Challenges Cancer*. (Note: These excerpts have been edited for translation purposes.)

- **Fifty-seven-year-old male, lung cancer (epidermoid carcinoma) stage IV**

The subject was diagnosed as stage IV and refused chemotherapy. The first cancer was diagnosed in 1985, as colloid carcinoma. By 1989, it had metastasized to the lung with a tumor size of 1.5 cm and 3.8 cm. The subject began 100 mg of MD fraction on a daily basis, but unfortunately died sixty months later (1994). However, the subject had shown improvement and the cancer diagnosis had improved to stage III-A before his passing away. After administration of MD fraction and tablets, 3.8 cm tumor shrank to 3 cm and the smaller cancer disappeared completely. However, his cancer had metastasized to the lymph nodes.

- **Forty-seven-year-old female, lung cancer with metastasis to the liver (hepatocellular carcinoma) stage II**

From 1994, the subject had received 80 $mg/m^2$ of Cisplatin (CDDP) a total of four times, but was switched to 50 mg of MD fraction and 4 g of tablets to be taken every day starting in 1995. After 2.5 years (1997), IL-2 production was increased to 2.2-fold by maitake administration, and we could not identify any liver tumor. By 1999, there was no evidence of any growth of the liver.

- **Fifty-four-year-old male, liver cancer (hepatocellular carcinoma) stage III ($T_3$, $N_1$, $M_0$)**

This patient had been treated with percutaneous ethanol injection (PEIT) and Adriamycin (ADM: 20 mg) injection since 1995, but finally refused this treatment because of the minimal effectiveness and severe side effects of ADM. He was then administered 40 mg of MD fraction and 5 g of maitake tablets per day along with five PEIT injections. After one year, the level of bilirubin reduced to 1.6 mg/dL from 3.2 mg/dL, and also albumin decreased from 3.1 mg/dL to 1.9 mg/dL. Also, the value of $CD4^+$ cell and IL-2 production were potentiated to 1.7 times and 1.4-fold, respectively.

Meanwhile, T factor changed from 3 to 0.

[Note: In Stage III details above, T factor 3 means that cancer diameter is greater than 4 cm. N factor 1 means that the cancers metastasized to one cancer site. $M_0$ means that there is no metastatis.]

- **Forty-five-year-old female, liver cancer (hepatocellular carcinoma) stage III**

This subject was diagnosed with stage III cancer with a serum bilirubin of 3.2 mg/dL, albumin of 2.1 g/dL, and prothrombin activation of 43 percent before treatment with maitake. She had been receiving trans-catheter arteial embolization (TAE) 10 mL of lipiodol and had four treatments of ADM, which were ineffective. She was then later switched to treatment with Cis Platin, which had to be stopped due to serious side effects. Then in January 1996, she began 100 mg of MD fraction and 4 g of maitake tablets along with 100 mg of 5-FU each day. As of September 1997, improved values were seen as bilirubin of 2.1, albumin 3.0, and prothrombia activation was improved to 72.2 percent. Since February 1998, the subject has been receiving only maitake products, and her diagnosis is now stage I.

- **Fifty-six-year-old male, liver cancer (hepatocellular carcinoma) stage IV**

Nine years ago, the subject was diagnosed with lung cancer (epidemoid carcinoma) and half of left lung was removed. The surgery was followed by chemotherapy. By 1994, the cancer had spread to the liver. The subject was then administered 150 mg of MD fraction and 6 g of maitake tablets per day. In 1999, his value of IL-2 production was enhanced to 1.7 times, and counts of $CD4^+$ cell also were increased 1.3-fold; however, the cancer tumor did not change.

- **Forty-one-year-old female, breast cancer (intraductal carcinoma) stage III**

$ER^+$ (Estrogen receptor positive) was observed in this patient who had a growth of 2.4 cm by 0.7 cm. In 1996, she had surgery to remove two of the solid cancers and then started the 10 mg of anti-estrogen (TAM) and 100 mg of 5-FU. In 1997, a cancer recurrence with a size of 1.3 cm was found in the lung. The subject was then started on 125 mg of MD fraction and 4 g of tablets every day for twenty months. In 1999, it was confirmed that the lung cancer had disappeared. While using maitake, IL-2 production and $CD4^+$ cell count were increased to 1.5 and 1.3 times, respectively.

Dr. Nanba states that "These small and non-random trials indicated to us that maitake MD fraction has the ability to suppress cancers of the lung, liver, and breast. MD fraction stimulates the immune system of patients with cancer as shown in Table 5.2 on page 28. Though the data is preliminary, the results of limited clinical studies based on MD fraction suggest the potential of healing and preventing cancer."[23]

MaitakeGold 404® appears to be most effective against breast, prostate, liver, and lung cancers. To date, it has been less effective against bone, blood, and brain cancers.

| TABLE 5.2. IMPROVEMENT ACTIVITIES OF MAITAKE IN VARIOUS CANCERS | | | | |
|---|---|---|---|---|
| | IL-2 Production | | Count of CD4+ Cell | |
| | Before | After | Before | After |
| Liver cancer (9 patients)* (Hepatocellular carcinoma) | 1.00 | 1.29 | 1.00 | 1.42 |
| Lung cancer (8 patients)* (Epidermoid carcinoma) | 1.00 | 1.37 | 1.00 | 1.51 |
| Leukemia (3 patients)* | 1.00 | 0.83 | 1.00 | 0.74 |

*\* Average values of patients*

## RECOMMENDED DOSAGE OF MAITAKEGOLD 404®

MaitakeGold 404® is available in both liquid and capsule form. The recommended dosage is 0.5 to 1 mg of MD fraction per kilogram of body weight per day. This level represents the therapeutic dosage recommended for people with cancer or who need substantial immune support (for example, those fighting infection). For maintenance or general support, the recommended dosage is 5–15 mg of the MD fraction daily. For best results, take MaitakeGold 404® twenty minutes before meals or on an empty stomach.

| TABLE 5.3. SUGGESTED DAILY DOSE OF MAITAKEGOLD 404® | | | |
|---|---|---|---|
| Weight | Total Daily Dose | Weight | Total Daily Dose |
| 70–79 lbs | 15–35 mg | 160–169 lbs | 36–76 mg |
| 80–89 lbs | 18–40 mg | 170–179 lbs | 38–81 mg |
| 90–99 lbs | 20–44 mg | 180–189 lbs | 40–85 mg |
| 100–109 lbs | 22–49 mg | 190–199 lbs | 43–90 mg |
| 110–119 lbs | 24–53 mg | 200–209 lbs | 45–94 mg |
| 120–129 lbs | 27–58 mg | 210–219 lbs | 47–99 mg |
| 130–139 lbs | 29–63 mg | 220–229 lbs | 49–103 mg |
| 140–149 lbs | 31–67 mg | 230–239 lbs | 52–108 mg |
| 150–159 lbs | 34–72 mg | 240–249 lbs | 54–112 mg |

## SAFETY

MaitakeGold 404® extract is produced using a special type of organic maitake mushroom and is extracted without the use of harsh solvents such as acetone, methane, or hexane. It also contains no preservatives, alcohol, yeast, sugar, animal products, or artificial colors or flavors. It has a remarkable safety record with data showing it to be nontoxic. In a small percentage of cases, it may cause loose stools that can be alleviated by cutting down on the dosage.

It can be used by children with a reduced dosage (half to quarter adult dose) with medical supervision.

People who have had organ transplants and are on immunosuppressive medications should not use this product without the consent of their supervising physician.

# 6. Additional Medicinal Uses of Maitake

Like most natural products, MaitakeGold 404® exerts a complex and multifactorial set of actions that make it useful for other applications. Some of the potential uses of MaitakeGold 404® include the treatment of fatigue, high blood pressure, liver disease, and HIV. Maitake's diverse action makes it a potential therapy for many conditions.

## CANDIDA

MaitakeGold 404® can be a beneficial supplement for those with chronic candida infection. Overgrowth of this fungus is associated with a multitude of possible conditions including fatigue, depression, irritable bowel syndrome, and several others. An inefficient immune system may be an underlying cause of the candida overgrowth. Some practitioners hesitate to recommend the ingestion of medicinal mushroom extracts for candida-related problems, fearing that a fungal extract could exacerbate overgrowth of the candida. This may be true of consuming mushrooms as a food but does not apply to MaitakeGold 404®, a purified extract. Doctors who prescribe it for patients suffering from candida report favorable results.

## CHRONIC FATIGUE SYNDROME

MaitakeGold 404® is a formula considered by many practitioners to be effective for ameliorating symptoms of chronic fatigue syndrome. Maitake's immunopotentiating and adaptogenic effect may help to resolve underlying immune dysfunction often seen with this condition.

## HIGH BLOOD PRESSURE

As with shiitake and reishi mushrooms, maitake has been shown in human and animal studies to reduce blood pressure. Scott Gerson, M.D., Assistant Clinical Professor at New York Medical College in the Department of Community and Preventive Medicine in New York City, has done considerable research on maitake with hypertensive patients and has found a remarkably high rate of favorable response in six-month trials.[24,25,26,27,28]

## HIGH CHOLESTEROL AND TRIGLYCERIDES

Some studies have found that maitake has a beneficial effect on cholesterol and triglyceride levels. For example, one study found that maitake-fed rats experienced significant and lasting reductions in serum cholesterol and triglyceride levels.[29]

## CONSTIPATION

Maitake has been found by Dr. Nanba and his researchers to relieve constipation.[30] Presumably, this is accomplished through a stimulation of bile flow from the liver and gallbladder that in turn stimulates bowel movements.

## HEPATITIS AND LIVER AILMENTS

In 1994, Chinese researchers studied the effects of an extract of maitake on thirty-two people with chronic hepatitis B. This randomized controlled study found the recovery rate in the maitake group to be 72 percent and 57 percent for the control group. Blood studies showed the conversion from a positive hepatitis B antigen to negative was 44 percent in the maitake group and 12 percent in the control group. Liver enzyme readings were also more positive in the maitake group.[31]

## HUMAN IMMUNODEFICIENCY VIRUS (HIV)

In the late 1980s, researchers found that oral doses of the maitake D fraction enhanced helper T cells. This brought questions about D fraction's ability to help people who have HIV, where helper T cell function is suppressed and the patient has weakened immunity. In November 1991, the National Cancer Institute found that a sulfated maitake fraction was active in a preliminary anti-HIV drug-screening test. The maitake compound was shown to have antiviral activity. It was, however, not considered a promising treatment due to concerns over toxicity.

However, a 2000 study by Dr. Nanba and his colleagues looked at the effect of MaitakeGold 404® extract on people with HIV. This study looked at the effects of 6 grams of tablets or 20 mg of purified MD fraction together with 4 grams of tablets per day for 360 days on thirty-five HIV-positive people. Researchers monitored T helper cell (CD4+) counts, viral load measure, symptoms of HIV infection, status of secondary disease, and the HIV in-fected individual's sense of well-being. The effects on T-helper cell count and viral load varied. However, some 85 percent of respondents reported an increased sense of well-being with regard to various symptoms and secondary diseases caused by HIV. Researchers concluded that "the active ingredients of maitake have significant healing and preventative potential in HIV-responders by stimulating the immune system." Interestingly, even though different immune cell activities were increased, there was no increase in HIV replication in CD4+ cells.[32] Thus, at this point in time, MaitakeGold 404® is one of the few natural substances to have shown safety and possible benefit for those with HIV infection.

MaitakeGold 404® may also hold promise for HIV-infected individuals who develop the skin cancer Kaposi's sarcoma. For example, Dr. David Hughes, with a private practice in San Bernardino, California, states: "A mixed liquid of MD fraction and the drug DSMO is effective against Kaposi's sarcoma." He found that applying the mixed fluid on the affected area four times a day for several days shrank the tumor.[33]

## WEIGHT LOSS

Maitake has been shown in both animal and human studies to help with weight loss. It has been shown to improve fat metabolism among maitake-fed rats.[34] More important, a clinical study on thirty overweight people found maitake supplementation resulted in weight loss. In this study, researchers gave maitake tablets equal to 200 grams of fresh maitake daily for two months. Subjects made no changes to their diet and all lost weight. Average weight loss was seven to thirteen pounds and one person lost approximately twenty-six pounds. The only side effect noted by a few patients was slightly looser stools.[35]

## FOR PETS

Animals have immune systems very similar in function to that of humans. Pet owners and veterinarians are now realizing the benefits of nontoxic supplements such as maitake for optimizing health and the complementary treatment of disease. MaitakeGold 404® can also be used for pets that require immune support, such as in the case of cancer or other immune-related matters as deemed appropriate by a veterinarian. Similar to my recommendation for humans, one can also give their pet maitake as a daily supplement to prevent breakdown of the immune system. For pets, an appropriate dosage would be 10 mg for animals ten to thirty pounds and 20 mg for animals thirty to seventy pounds.

# Conclusion

For centuries, both physicians and ordinary people of Japan have held maitake in high esteem. Today, current scientific research has brought to life the many remarkable healing properties of this medicinal mushroom. The special MD fraction in MaitakeGold 404® extract is the culmination of decades of scientific research and is the form most recommended as a preventative and therapeutic supplement. It is proving to be not only a valuable supplement for immunity but also for cellular protection and as an adaptogen of the immune system. MaitakeGold 404® extract remains a premier nutritional supplement in the battle against cancer. It works to harness the power of the immune system, an essential component of cancer prevention and treatment. I am also excited about the use of MaitakeGold 404® extract for people with HIV. It is one of the few natural substances shown to exhibit therapeutic activity while not accelerating the replication of HIV. Maitake should be a strong consideration for those with acute and chronic viral infections as seen with hepatitis and some cases of chronic fatigue syndrome. Lastly, it should be used as an everyday supplement for optimal immune function and vitality.

MaitakeGold 404® is a unique and patented strain of organically grown maitake (*Grifola frondosa*) with which all of Dr. Nanba's studies have been conducted. All of his research on the maitake D fraction and maitake MD fraction have been from this proprietary strain of maitake mushroom extract as cultivated by the Yukuguni Maitake Company of Japan. Maitake MD fraction as found in MaitakeGold 404® is the only product Dr. Nanba's endorses and recommends.

The research continues on MaitakeGold 404®. A study is scheduled to begin at a major North American cancer research center in 2002. This trial in breast cancer patients involves three stages of testing. First, MaitakeGold 404® will be tested for its compatibility with chemotherapy agents. Next, healthy volunteers will be given this extract to further research its bioavailability and effect against breast cancer cells (MCF-7) in tissue culture. A third stage of research will look at the benefits of MaitakeGold 404® when used with chemotherapy to eliminate tumors.

This research will hopefully help MaitakeGold 404® to become an accepted cancer therapy in North America.

# Resources

The companies listed below utilize in their products the authentic Maitake-Gold 404® developed by Dr. Hiroaki Nanba and used in his extensive body of research. Contact information is provided to enable you to obtain further information about their products. None of the manufacturers and distributors listed below has had any connection with the production of this book. Rather, we list these companies because we believe their products to be effective and of high quality. Please be aware that this information is subject to change.

**Carotec, Inc.**
P.O. Box 9919
Naples, FL 34101
800-522-4279
www.carotec.com

**Carrington Laboratories**
Aloeceuticals/Caraloe
2001 Walnut Hill Lane
Irving, TX 75038
800-444-ALOE (2563)
www.carringtonlabs.com

**DaVinci Laboratories
of Vermont**
20 New England Drive
Essex Junction, VT 05453
800-325-1776
www.davincilabs.com

**Doctor's A-Z**
Distributed by Great American
Health Products, Wholesale
Distributors
P.O. Box 2672
Fargo, ND 58108-2672
800-437-2733

**FoodScience of Vermont**
20 New England Drive
Essex Junction, VT 05453
800-874-9444
www.foodscienceofvermont.com

**Gaia Herbs, Inc.**
108 Island Ford Road
Brevard, NC 28712
800-831-7780
www.gaiaherbs.com

## HomeCure Inc.

P.O. Box 41420
Mesa, AZ 85274-1420
800-559-CURE (2873)
www.Homecure.com

## JHS Natural Products

P.O. Box 50398
Eugene, OR 97405
888-330-4691
www.jhsnp.com / www.jhspro.com

## Langel Enterprise & Associates

360 East Randolph Street, Suite 504
Chicago, IL 60601
888-292-9365
www.langelenterprises.com

## Life Extension Foundation

800-544-4440 • 954-761-9199
www.LifeExtension.com

## MegaFood

8 Bowers Road
Derry, NH 03038
800-848-2542
www.megafood.com

## Mushroom Science

1025 Conger Street, #6
Eugene, OR 97402
888-283-6583
www.MushroomScience.com

## Natural Factors Nutritional Products

1111 80th Street, SW
Everrett, WA 98203
425-513-8800, ext. 3
www.naturalfactors.com

## Natural Factors Nutritional Products (Canada)

1550 United Blvd.
Coquitlam, BC V3K 6Y7

## Nutri-Active/GNC

9 Ubi Crescent
Singapore 408572
Tel: (65) 6285-6778
Fax: (65) 6285-1579
www.nutri-active.org

## Swanson Health Products

P.O. Box 2803
Fargo, ND 58108-2803
800-437-4148
www.swansonvitamins.com

## Thorne Research Inc.

P.O. Box 25
Dover, ID 83825
800-228-1966
www.Thorne.com

## Threshold Enterprises, Ltd.

Planetary Formulas
P.O. Box 533
Soquel, CA 95073
800-606-6226
www.planetaryformulas.com

## Zand Herbal Formulas

1441 West Smith Road
Ferndale, WA 98248
800-232-4005
www.zand.com

For an updated listing of companies that carry MaitakeGold 404® as well as further information, visit the website www.maitakegold.com.

# Notes

1. American Cancer Society website 2001. www.cancer.org, June 2001.

2. Hobbs C. *Medicinal Mushrooms.* Loveland, CO: Interweave Press Inc., 1996, p.110.

3. Nanba H and Kumar P. *The Therapeutics of Maitake Mushroom in Japan.* Kobe, Japan: New Editions Health World, 1995, p. 21.

4. Mizuno T. Zhuang C. "Maitake, *Grifola frondosa*: Pharmacological effects." *Food Rev Int* 11(1):135–149 (1995).

5. Nanba H. "Activity of Maitake D fraction to Inhibit Carcinogenesis and Metastasis." *New York Academy of Sciences,* vol. 768, p. 243 (September 30, 1995).

6. Nanba H. "Activity of Maitake D fraction to Inhibit Carcinogenesis and Metastasis". *New York Academy of Sciences,* vol. 768, p. 243–245 (September 30, 1995).

7. Nanba H, Kubo K. Antitumor substance extracted from Grifola. U.S. Patent 5,854,404, issued December 29, 1998.

8. ibid.

9. Nanba H. Presented at the 3rd International Conference on Mushroom Biology and Mushroom Products in Sydney, Australia (October 1999).

10. Nanba H. *Maitake Challenges Cancer.* Kobe, Japan: Socio Health Group, 1998.

11. Hobbs, C. *Medicinal Mushrooms.* Loveland, CO: Interweave Press Inc., 1996, p. 110.

12. U.S. Environmental Protection Agency, 1987–1994 Toxic Release Inventory National Report. Washington, D.C: Office of Toxic Substances.

13. Nanba H. "Effect of maitake D fraction on cancer prevention." *Ann NY Acad Sci* 1997;833:204–07.

14. Kurashings S, et al. "Effects of Lentinus edodes, *Grifola frondosa,* and Pleurotus ostreus administration on cancer outbreak, and activities of macrophages and lymphocytes in mice treated with a carcinogen N-butyl-N-butanolninitrosamine." *Immunopharmacol Immunotoxicol,* 19(2):175-83. (May 1997).

15. Nanba H. "Activity of maitake D fraction to inhibit carcinogenesis and metastasis." *Ann NY Acad Sci* 1995;768:243–45.

16. Adachi K, Nanba H, Kuroda H. "Potentiation of host-mediated antitumor activity in mice by beta-glucan obtained from *Grifola frondosa* (maitake)." *Chem Pharm Bull* 1987;35: 262–70.

17. Lovy A, Knowles B, Labbe R, Nolan L. "Activity of edible mushrooms against the growth of human T4 leukemic cancer cells, HeLa cervical cancer cells, and Plasmodium falciparum." *J Herbs, Spices, Medicinal Plants,* 1998.

18. Nanba H. *Maitake Challenges Cancer.* Kobe, Japan: Socio Health Group, 1998.

19. Nanba H. "Maitake D fraction: Healing and preventive potential for cancer." *J Orthomol Med* 1997;12(1):43–49.

20. Nanba H. Presented at the 3rd International Conference on Mushroom Biology and Mushroom Products in Sydney, Australia (October 1999).

21. ibid.

22. ibid.

23. ibid.

24. Nanba H. and Kumar P. *The Therapeutics of Maitake Mushroom in Japan.* Kobe, Japan: New Editions Health World, 1995, p.33.

25. Kabir Y, et al. "Effect of shiitake (*Lentinus edodes*) and maitake (*Grifola frondosa*) mushrooms on blood pressure and plasma lipids of spontaneously hypertensive rats." *J Nutr Sci Vitaminol* 1987;33(5):341–46.

26. Kabir Y, Kimura S. "Dietary mushrooms reduce blood pressure in spontaneously hypertensive rats (SHR)." *J Nutr Scir Vitaminol* 1989;35(1):91–94.

27. Kabir Y, Hoshino T, Komai M, Kimura S. "Histopathological changes in spontaneously hypertensive rats after feeding shiitake (Lentinus edodes) and maitake (*Grifola frondosa*) mushroom diets." *J Clin Biochem Nutr* 1989;6:187–93.

28. Adachi K, Nanba H, Otuska M, Kuroda H. "Blood pressure-lowering activity present in the fruit body of *Grifola frondosa* (maitake).": 1. *Chem Pharm Bull* 1988;36(3):1000–06.

29. Kubo K, Nanba H. "Anti-hyperliposis effect of maitake fruit body (*Grifola frondosa*)." 1. *Biol Pharm Bull* 1997 Jul;20(7):781–85.

30. Nanba H. *Maitake Challenges Cancer.* Kobe, Japan: Socio Health Group, 1998.

31. Wu S, Zou D, Hans S.H, et al. Therapeutic effect of Grifola polysaccharides in chronic hepatitis B (abstract P-18). In: International Symposium on Production and Products of Lentinus Mushroom, Programme and Abstract, Qinggyuan, Zhejiang Province, China: International Society for Mushroom Science, Committee on Science Asian Region, Qingyuan County of Government, Shejiang Province, China, 1994.

32. Nanba H, Kodama N, Schar D, Turner D. "Effects of maitake (*Grifola frondosa*) glucan in HIV-infected patients," *Mycoscience* 2000;41:293–95.

33. Mavlit G, Ishii Y, Patt Y, et al. "Local xenogenic graft-vs-host reaction: a practical assessment of T-cell function among cancer patients." *Journal of Immunology* 1979; 123(5):2185–2188.

34. Yokota M. Observatory trial of anti-obesity activity of maitake mushroom (*Grifola frondosa*). Anshin (Tokyo) July 1992;202–03.

35. ibid.

# Index

# About the Author

Mark Stengler, N.D., serves on a committee for the Yale University Complementary Medicine Outcomes Research Project. He is the author of several books, including *The Natural Physician's Healing Therapies; Your Vital Child; Nature's Virus Killers;* and *Your Menotype, Your Menopause.* He practices as a family naturopathic doctor in La Jolla, California.

His website is www.thenaturalphysician.com.